Medicine for kids

Jibran Naseer MD

CONTENTS

Introduction

Since the authors children were young, he would tell his kids bedtime stories of the patients he had seen that day. They found them fascinating, and thus grew his idea to teach young kids about common medical problems and their treament. He would like to share some of his experiences with you.

1. EAR CLEANING

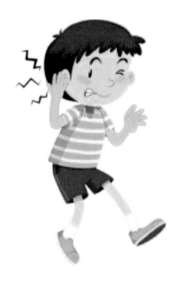

If an insect sneaks into your ear without you noticing,, theres no need to panic!

There is a very easy solution to get out of this unfortunate turn of events. You will simply need to tilt your head to the side and put ten drops of oil into the affected ear canal. Wait for at least ten minutes and then bring your head back to straight. This will get the insect out, and you can then use earbuds to get the excess oil out of your ear.

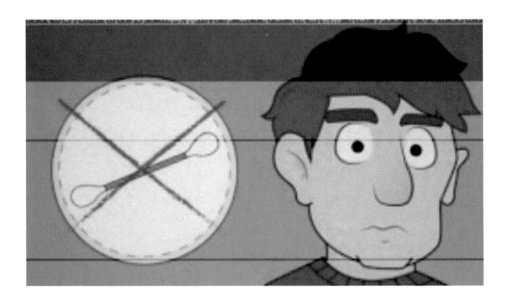

Fun Fact:

Your ears can clean themselves with the help of many tiny hair like structures. By trying to clean the inside of the ears you can actually cause impaction of the ear wax.

The ear has the smallest bone in the body!

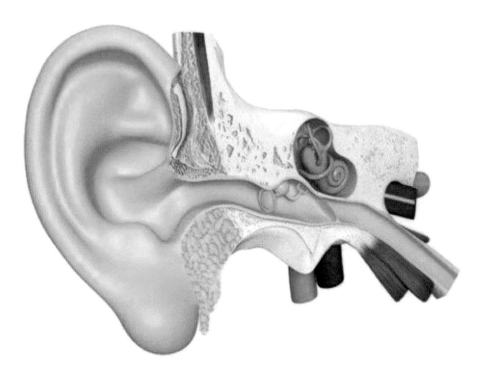

2. EYE INJURY

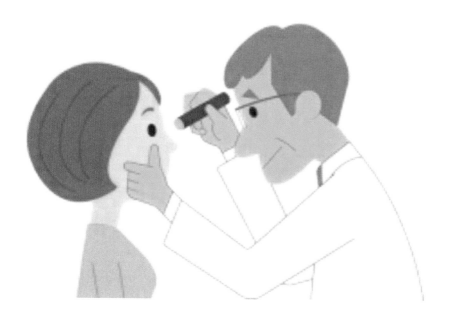

When a group of children are playing together, getting a blow of a metal object in the eyes is not a very rare occurrence. If you get hit in the eye with a metal object, you should immediately go home and apply some ice on the affected eye without applying much pressure. A piece of metal in the eye needs to be removed immediately as it can lead to scarring and affect your vision.

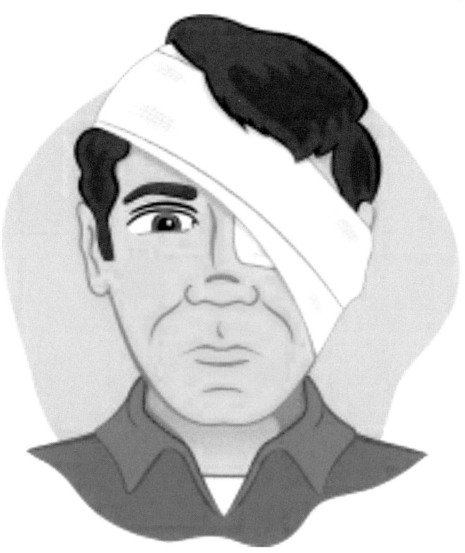

Fun Fact :

A metal piece can form a rust ring in the eye which can cause scarring and affect vision.

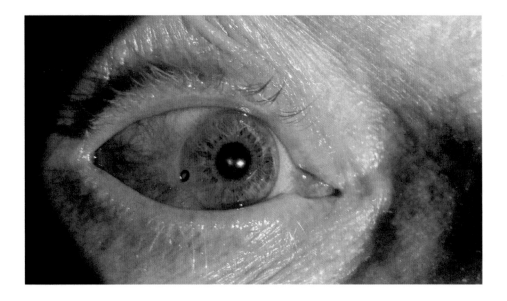

3. PINK EYE

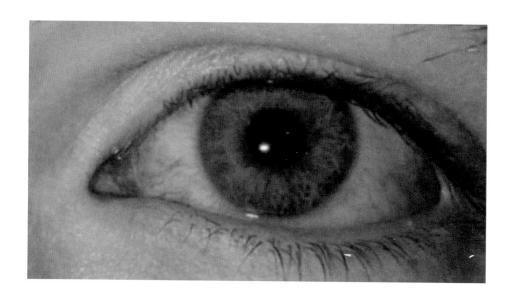

"Pink eye" is something that we all are familiar with. It is mostly caused by a virus. If you have gotten pink eye, it is best to keep your distance from others as it is quite **contagious**. It will cause itching, redness and watery eyes.

Wearing sunglasses and avoiding close contact with others helps reduce the spread. However, there is nothing to be alarmed about as pink eye generally cures on its own.

Fun Fact: Allergies can cause pink eye as well.

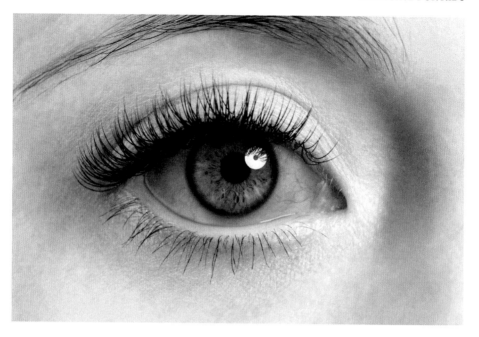

4. VOMITING & DIARRHEA

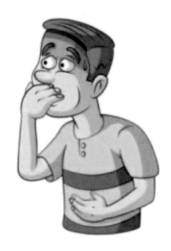

Vomiting and diarrhea can be quite messy! It is mostly caused by viruses that get carried into our gut with dirty hands. That is why it is very important that we wash our hands before we eat and do not let insects sit on our foods. These insects often sit on poop and carry the virus and other germs where ever they go. Because of the same reason, we should avoid eating roadside foods that remain in open air.

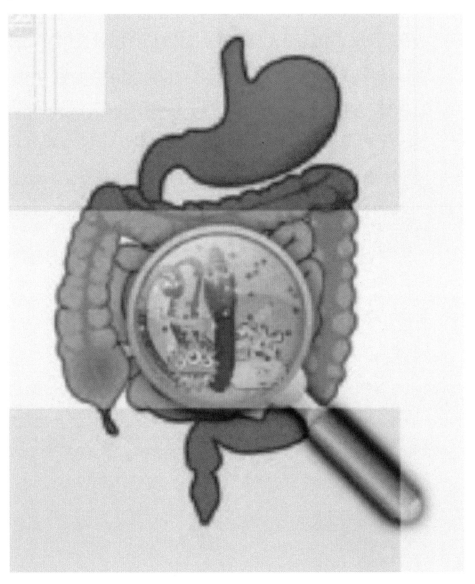

Fun Fact :

A lot of people do not use soap to wash their hands and only wash them for less than 6 seconds. Thats why the restrooms at restaurants have a sign on the mirror "Employees must wash their hands".

5. BACK PAIN

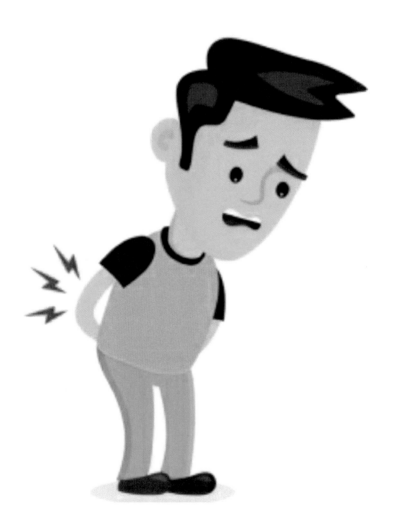

Back pain is something that one would not forget easily because of the intense pain it causes. Our back is made up of muscles, bones, nerves, and any of those can cause back pain. You can also have internal organs cause back pain, such kidney stones. Stretching exercises are very helpful for most backaches.

Fun Fact :

Humans and Giraffes
have the same amount of
vertebras in their necks.

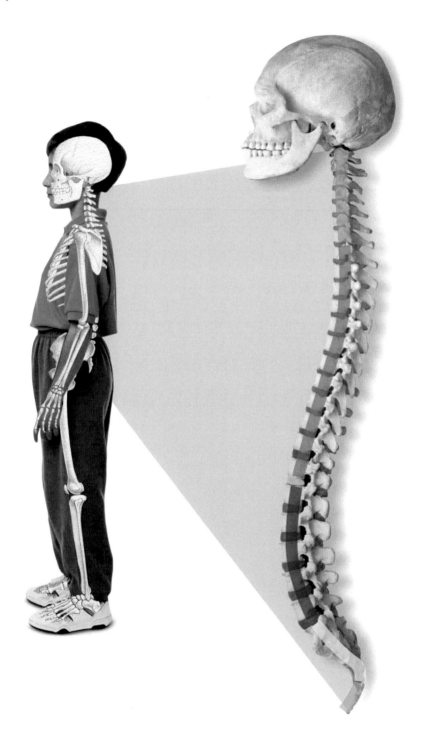

6. INFLUENZA

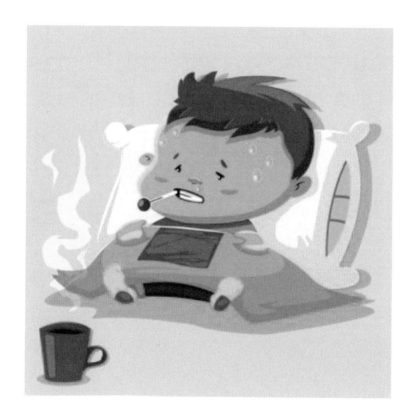

Every one has experienced getting the Flu. The Influenza Virus mutates quite rapidly and that is why vaccines often fail. The flu causes fever, chills, congestion and a lot of body aches. You should give your body a lot of rest and drink plenty of juice and water to ensure a speedy recovery.

Fun Fact :

The word influenza is Italian meaning "influence"
There are 3 different types of In-

fluenza virus, Influenza A, B & C but they have multiple strains.

7. FRACTURES

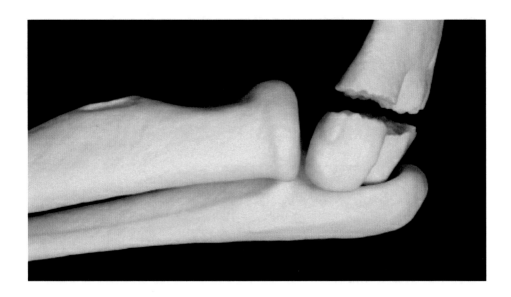

Fracturing your bones is not a rare occurrence. It can happen while

having a good game of foot-
ball or absent mindedly missing
your steps on the stairs. Though
it is very painful to go through a
broken bone, fractures heal completely within six weeks or so.
However, you must ensure that
you have proper casting and are
giving it enough rest.

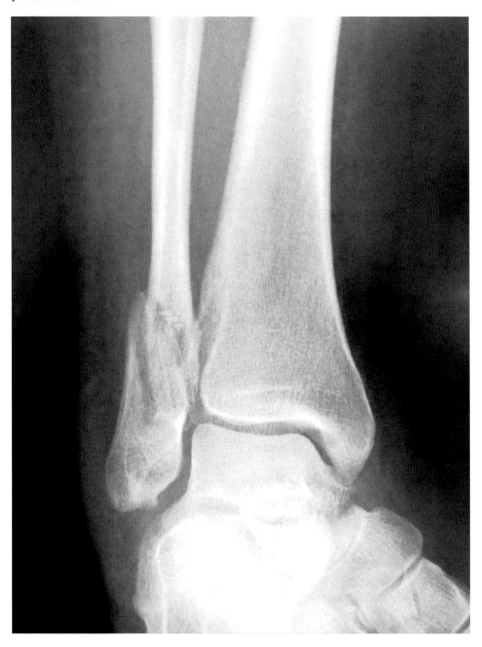

Fun Facts : A spiral or

twisted fracture of a bone
needs surgery to make sure
the bone can heal well.

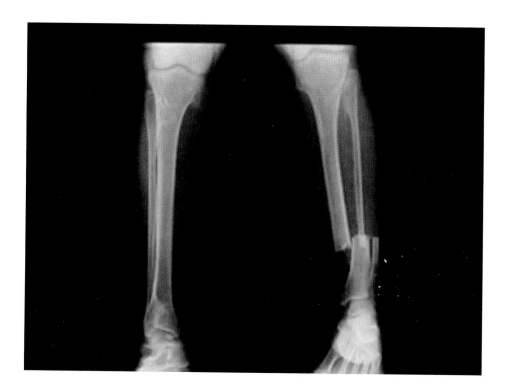

8. WOUNDS & SCARS

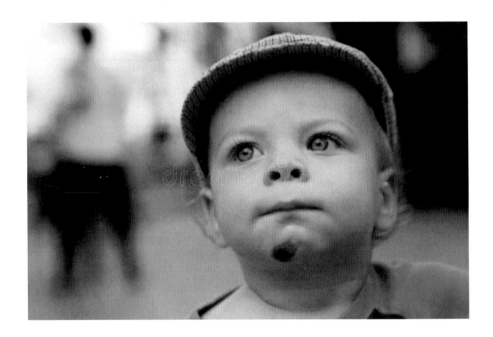

We are all familiar with the fact that all wounds leave a mark; no matter how small, there will be a scar for every wound you get. However, the scar formation process is quite long and generally takes about a year to fully form.

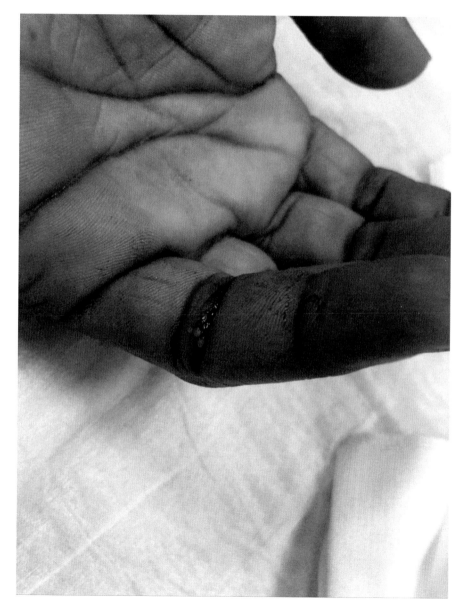

9. EYES & EARS

Human beings cannot hear all the sounds around them. We can only hear the sound waves having a frequency between 20 to 20,000 Hz. The most sensitive range for human hearing is 2000-5000 Hz.

Regarding the visibility of light, human eyes can discern the light that has a frequency between 405 to 790 THz.

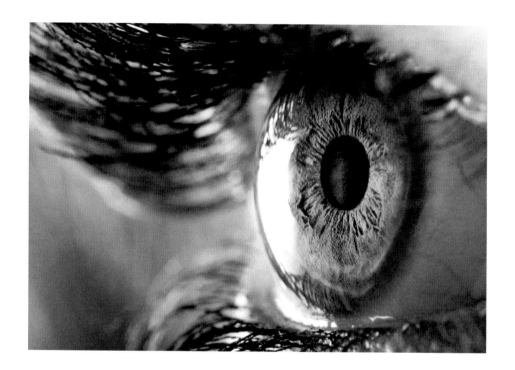

Fun Fact :

The human eye can only see a
tiny part of the electromagnetic
spectrum called the visible

light spectrum.
Many types of light like radio, X-rays, Gamma rays, Ultraviolet, infrared are invisible to human eyes.

10. ANIMAL BITES

Getting bitten by a rabid animal is something that almost everyone is quite scared of. The only way to confirm if the animal had rabies is through a brain biopsy. Wild animals can be carry rabies but even animals living in the cities like bats and dogs can have it.

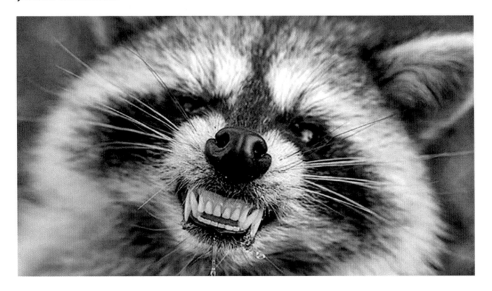

Fun Facts :

If you are bitten by a wild animal, you might need to get a series of 4 shots to prevent rabies. OUCH!

11. POOP

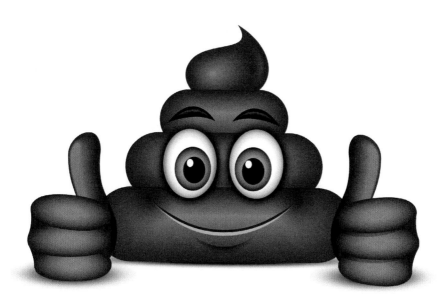

Did you know that **90% percent** of the your poop is made of bacteria. The remaining ten percent contains protein, water, fats and undigested foods. Having healthy pooping habits is as important as healthy eating habits!

Fun Facts :

Babies poop every time they eat. As we grow older it begins getting less frequent.

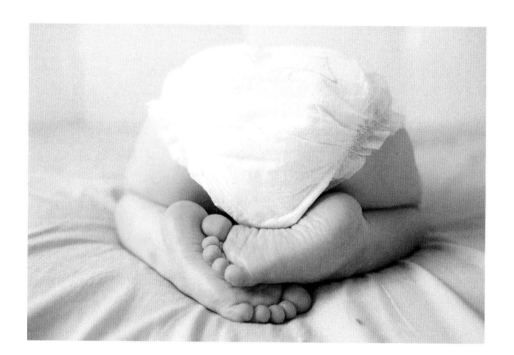

12. SKIN

Skin is the outer layer that covers our body like a blanket. It not only protects our insides but also has important functions to control out temperature, help us feel our surroundings and protect our body from infections.

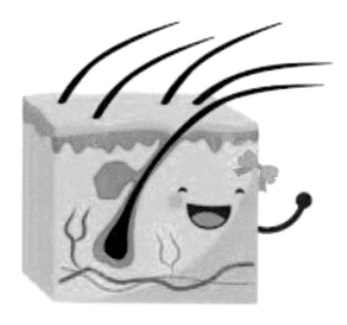

13. BRAIN

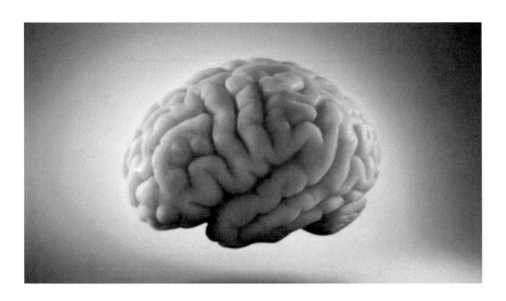

The human brain is a fascinating place, isn't it?

The brain is what holds it all

together, and all our thoughts and ideas have got their home in the brain. The human brain contains more than 80 billion cells or neurons that transmit information to different parts of our body. Neurons are the basic working unit of the brain. Our brain never sleeps and has a map of our whole body in it to control all the functions.

14. IMMUNE SYSTEM

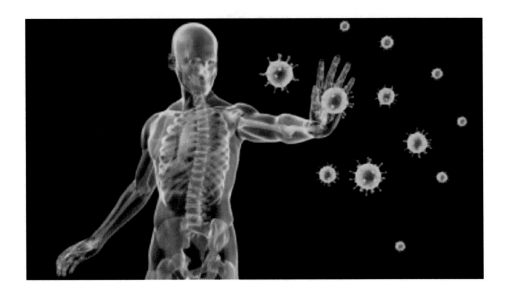

Our immune system is the

shield that protects us against the attack of different viruses and bacteria. A strong immune system can put up a good fight with any type of injury, infection and even cancer. One should eat healthy andexercise regulary to keep the immune system strong.

Fun Fact :

The immune system can detect any danger to our body and quickly send its soldiers called antibodies out to remove and kill the things causing damge to the body. But sometimes our own immune system can start fighting against our own body and destroy its cells.

15. LYME DISEASE

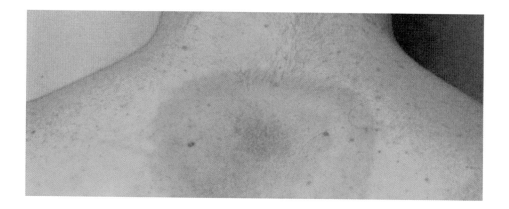

Black legged ticks carry the Lyme disease. These ticks mainly get bacteria from deer or mice. If you have been bitten by a black legged tick carrying the Lyme disease, then there is a rash called erythema migrans. The tick bites and gets full of blood and gets twice the size and it is very difficult to take it off the skin. The entire tick has to be removed from the skin.

Fun Fact :

Lyme disease can cause over 300 different symptoms.

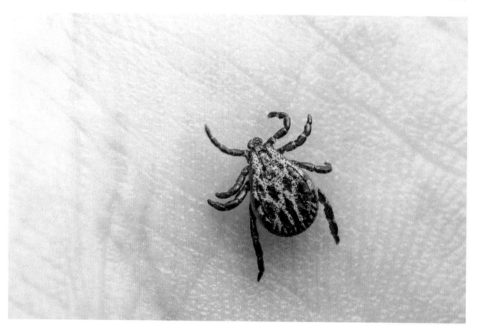

16. RINGWORM

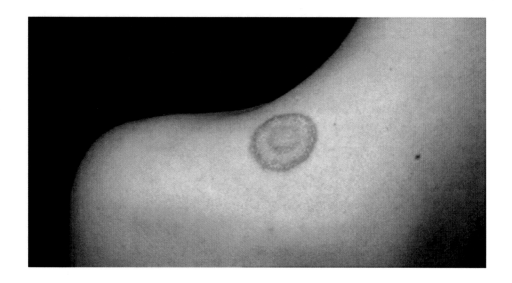

Ringworm is a very common skin infection and it is caused by a fungus. It is contagious and generally spreads by direct skin contact. The rash is itchy and makes a red ring. The fungus likes to grow in moist areas.

Fun Fact :

Ringworm gets its name from ring like, circular rash. Ringworm has NO worms in it.

17. SUBUNGUAL HEMATOMA

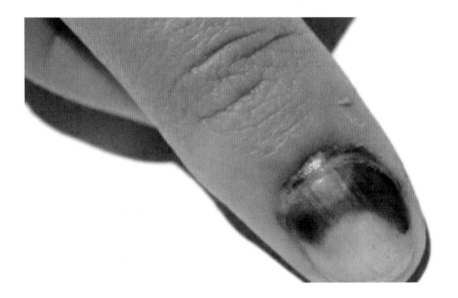

We often have been injured on our nails that has caused the nail to turn black. There is a medical term for this bleeding under the nail and it is called subungual hematoma. In order to make the pain better you have to drain out the blood.

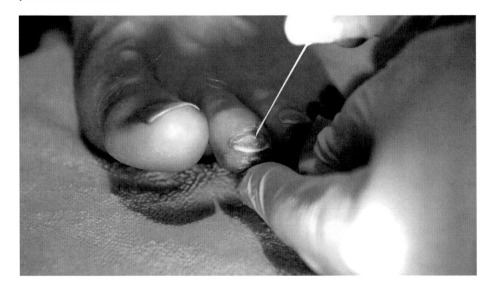

Fun Fact :

In case of emergency, you can drain the blood from under the nail by using a hot needle and making a hole in the nail. This should drain the blood and give quick relief of pain.

18. ABSCESS

An abscess is a pocket filled with pus. It is like a pimple but mostly under the skin. Besides antibiotics, it is important that the abscess is cut open to drain the pus. Sometimes you can place a piece of guaze or cloth in it to keep it open while it heals.

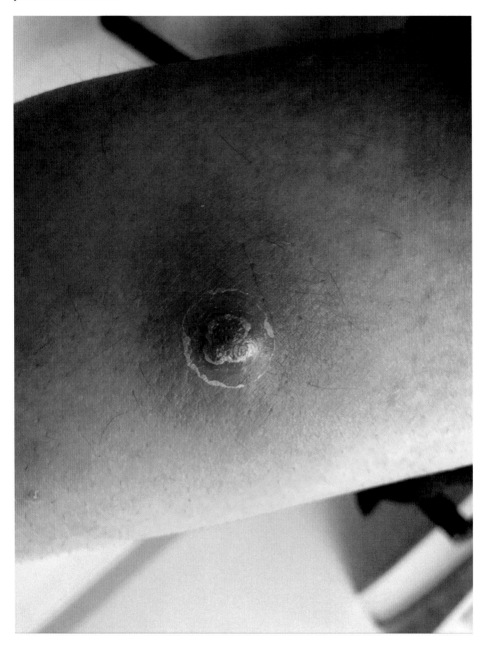

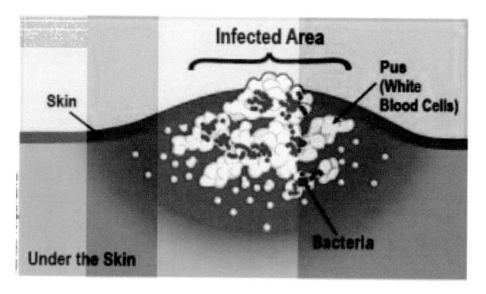

19. HONEY

Honey does not only taste yummy but it also has a number of health benefits as well. If you have burns or wound on your skin, honey can work well as an anti-inflammatory. It is also used for burns on the skin to reduce infection risks.

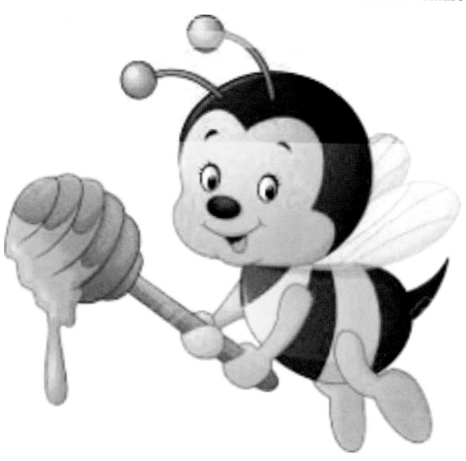

20. NOSEBLEEDS

Nosebleeds are something that a lot of people have encountered. One of the most basic reasons for nosebleeds is a change in the surrounding temperature. In case you get a nosebleed, you should pinch the tip of your nose tightly and lean forward for 10 to 15 minutes.

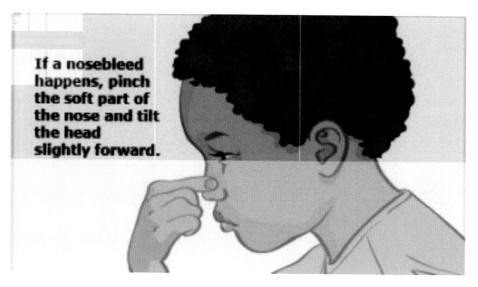

If a nosebleed happens, pinch the soft part of the nose and tilt the head slightly forward.

Fun Fact :

The majority of nose bleeds occur from the front of the nose known as "Little's Area"

21. BRONCHITIS

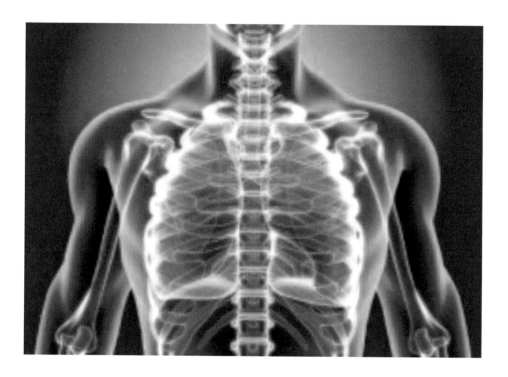

Bronchitis is the most common lung infection. It causes cough with mucus coming up from your chest. Most bronchitis is caused by viruses but it can take up to 3 weeks to resolve.

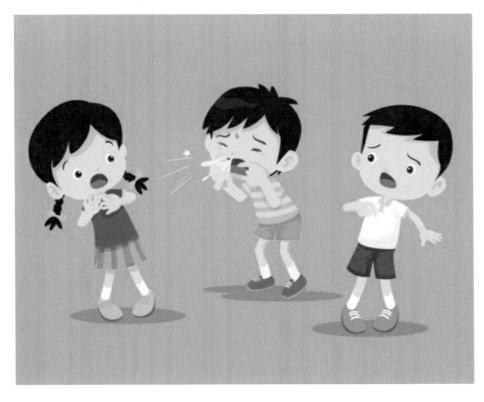

One of the best ways to avoid spreading germs when you are coughing is by doing a vampire

cough (coughing in your elbow)

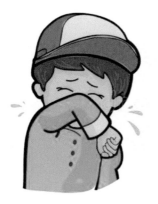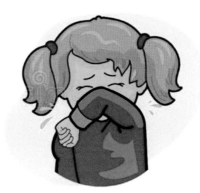

Fun Fact:

The left lung it smaller than the right lung to accomodate for the heart in the chest on the left side.

22. WARTS

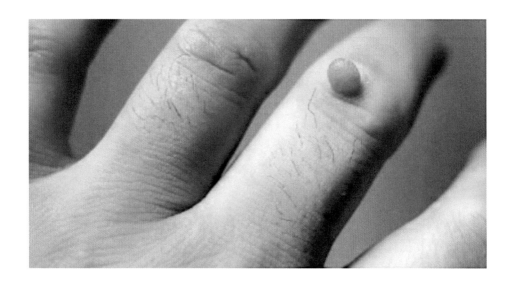

Warts are growths on your skin that are caused by a virus called the human papillomavirus.

There are over 60 types of this virus and some of them can cause skin warts. In order to treat them, they can be frozen by using an extremely cold so-lution called liquid nitrogen or they can be cut from the skin.

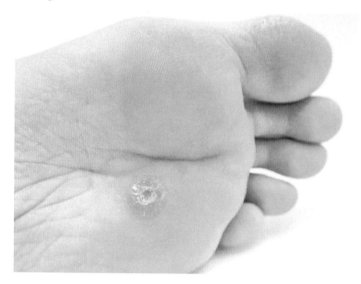

Fun Fact :

Warts are contagious with

close skin to skin contact!

23. BELL'S PALSY

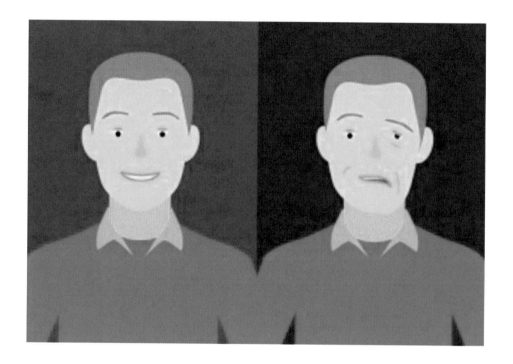

Bell's Palsy is a condition where

your face droops to one side. It is mostly related to a viral infection that causes inflammation of the Facial nerve that controls the muscle on that side of face and also the tears, taste, saliva production on that side.

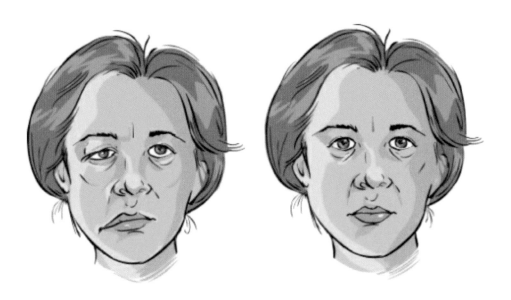

Fun Facts :

You have a hard time closing your affected eye completely or smile on the side of Bell's palsy.

24. HEIMLICH MANEUVER AND CHOKING

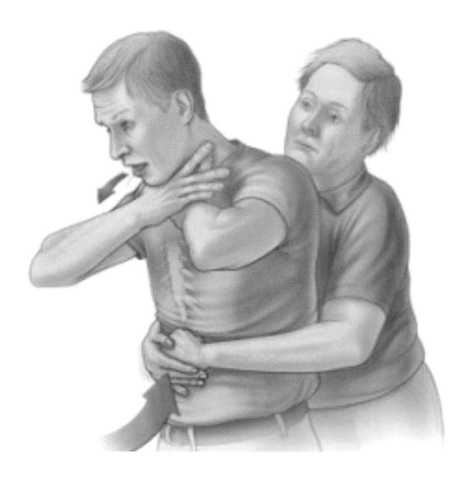

If someone is choking you must do the Heimlich maneuver to help that person. You hold the choking person from the back and place your fist over his/her navel. Then, grab your fist with your other hand and push it inward and upward until the choking is resolved and the person can breathe again.

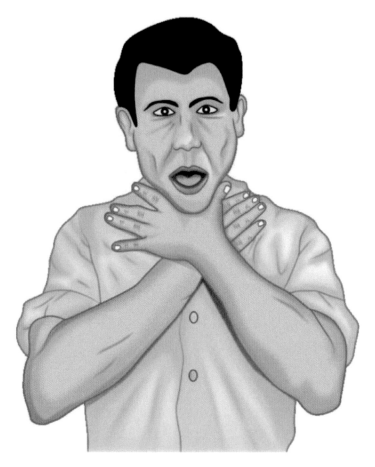

Fun Fact :

When someone is choking, they make the "Universal Choking sign"

25. TOENAIL FUNGUS

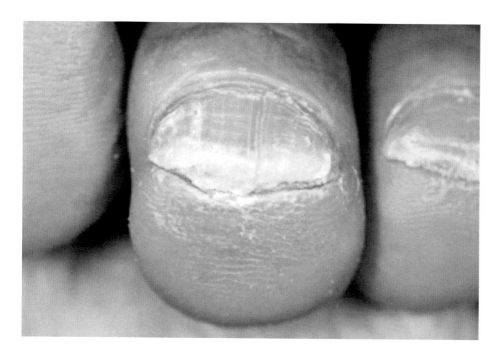

Toenail fungus is an
infection caused by
fungus and its medical

name is Onychomychosis (say that 5 times)

It might cause your nail to change its color, make nails loose and thicker. The same infection can cause athlete's foot infection between the toes with an itchy rash.

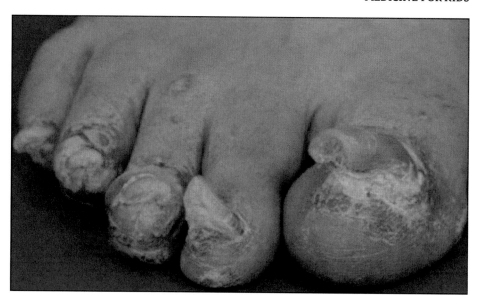

Fun Fact : A mixture of vinegar and water can be used as a home remedy to treat it.

26. MOSQUITO BITES

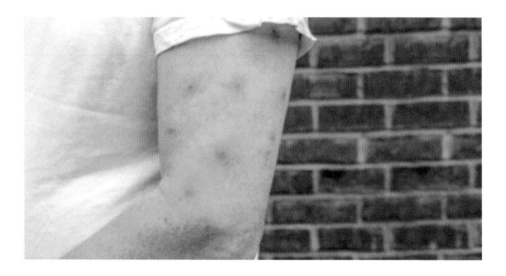

You might be familiar with

mosquito bites and the nuisance they are! While not all mosquitoes are carriers of harmful diseases, some can pose serious threats of causing diseases like Malaria. It is, therefore, better to remain safe from mosquito bites using mosquito repellants at home and keeping the surroundings of the house clean.

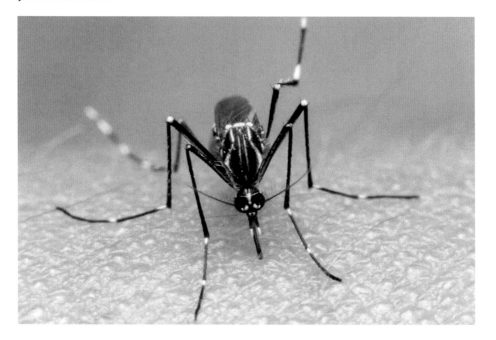

27. SKIN

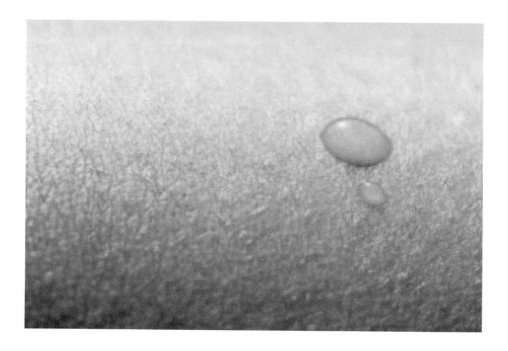

Skin covers the entire body and has multiple layers. The outer layer is known as the epidermis, next layer is dermis and it consists of dense connective tissues that has the hair follicles, blood vessels, sweat glands, and a number of other structures.

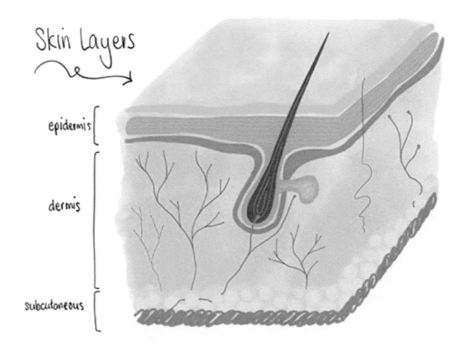

Skin Layers

epidermis

dermis

subcutaneous

Fun Fact : Skin is the largest organ of your body.

28. WHITEHEADS

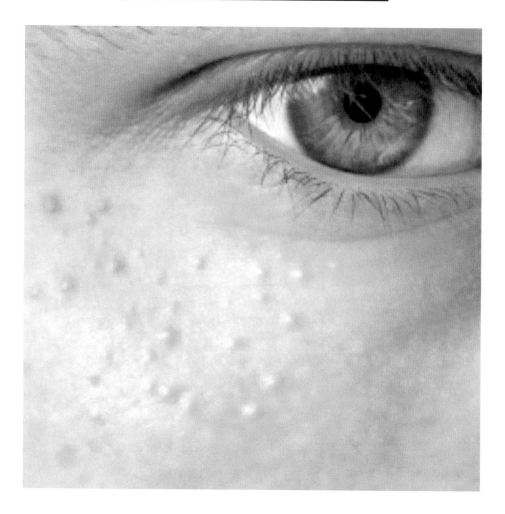

Whiteheads are quite a common occurrence and are mainly caused by clogged pores. The pores are actually oil glands in our skin that keeps our skin moist. Whiteheads can lead to acne as well. The best way to get rid of them is by gentle exfoliation.

29. BLACKHEADS

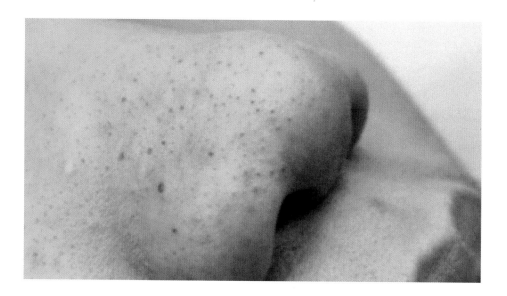

Blackheads occur due to unre-solved whiteheads.

If they remain open, they may

come into contact with oxygen in the air and lead to blackheads. You should also use a skin brush to brush off your skin. You can try a clay mask to cleanse your skin and free it of blackheads.

30. EAR WAX

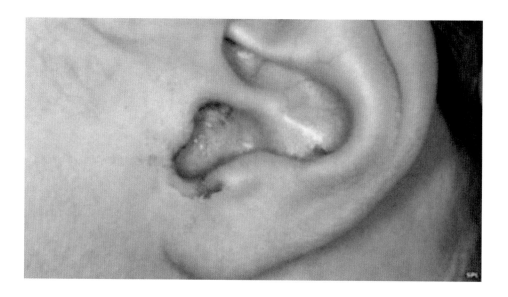

A waxy oil is produced inside our ears known as cerumen. The common name for it is earwax. This is naturally produced by the body to keep the ear safe from foreign objects. We are supposed to have some ear wax to protect our ears, however earwax can prove to be a problem for some people. Too much of it can cause hearing loss and sometimes pain.

Fun Fact : Excessive amounts of ear wax can be removed by washing the ears out and also using an instruement called Currette.

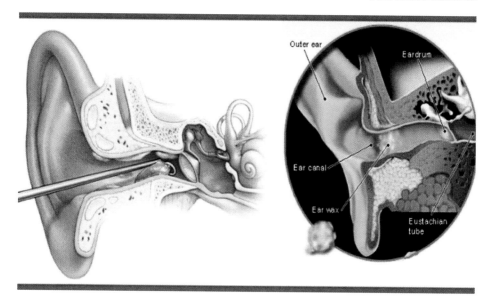

31. HEART

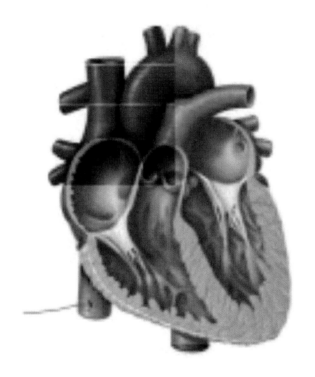

Everyone knows that it is the heart that keeps beating to keep us alive. Our heart is a muscular organ that has the size of a fist. Its position is just behind and on the slight left of the breastbone. The heart pumps blood throughout the network of veins and arteries that is known as the cardiovascular system.

ACTIVITY:

1. If you want to figure out the most beats your heart can do in a minute, the calculation is 220 minus your

age – so in your case, 220 minus nine equals 211 beats per minute, when you're exercising as hard as possible. For someone of my age, it's around 173 beats per minute.

2. To feel how hard your heart

works, try clenching and relaxing your fist 60 times in a minute. Hard work, right? And remember, your heart beats 60 times per minute, 60 minutes an hour, 24 hours a day, and 365 days per year. That would be 31,536,000 beats every year – if all we did was just sit still! Luckily, your heart does get to have a little rest in between every beat.

32. BONES

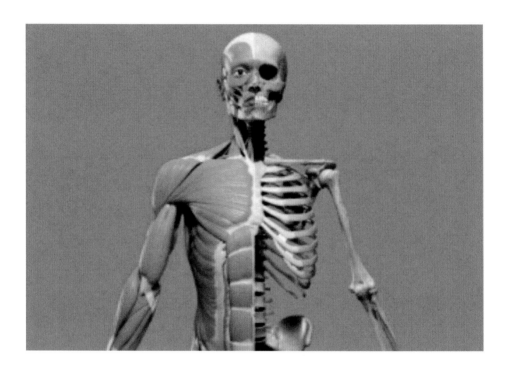

We know that the human body has 206 bones. However, the interesting fact here is that children have 300 bones at time of birth. As we age and the skeleton grows, the bones fuse together to make the 206 bones that the adults have. This fusion of the bones occurs later in life.

33. BORBORYGMI

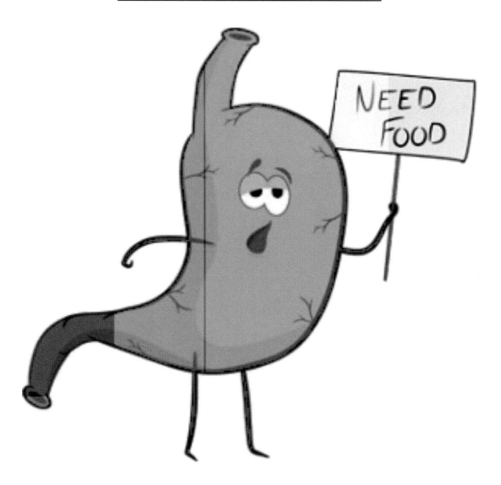

Everyone has experienced their stomach growling and making weird noises. It is a natural occurence and mainly happens due to the hunger. The medical term for this is borborygmi.

Next time this happens to you, say Borborygmi outoud so no one can hear your stomach growling.

34. TONGUE PRINTS

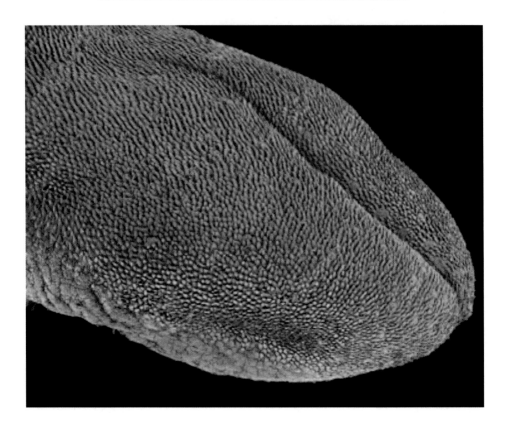

It is quite well known that fingerprints are unique to everyone but what a lot of people do not know is that tongue prints are unique s well! Even identical twins do not share the same tongue prints. Due to this uniqueness of the tongue prints, it has often been considered to use it as a potential tool for identification over the fingerprints.

35. PLATELETS

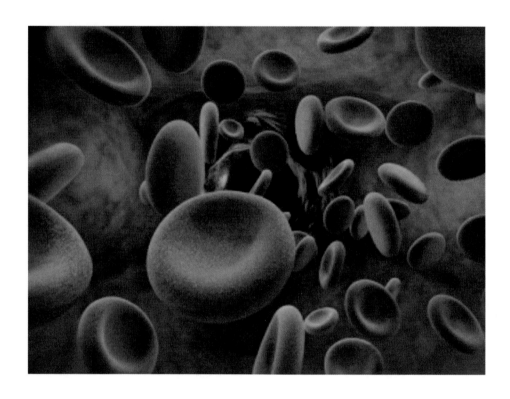

If you get a cut on your finger, it begins to bleed. Soon the body stops the bleeding! This happens when a clot forms at the area of the cut by blood cells called platelets. They help us from bleeding excessively and keep our body in a healthy state.

36. ANKLE SPRAINS

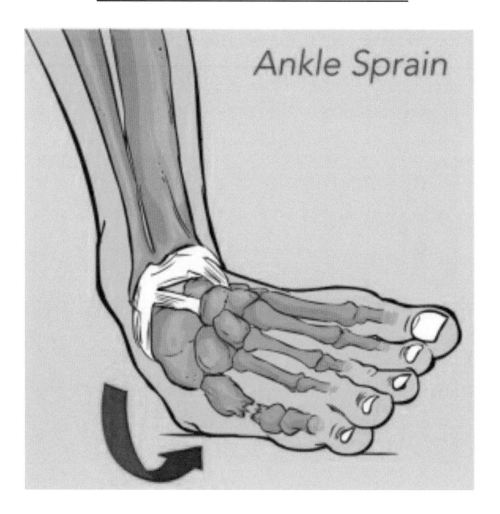

Rolling your ankle is very common. If you roll your ankle it will cause pain, swelling and make it difficult to walk on that foot and ankle. You will need to rest the ankle, elevate it to reduce swelling, ice it, and use compression. In an ankle sprain, ligaments are torn that help to keep the joints and bones in a place and are like rubber bands.

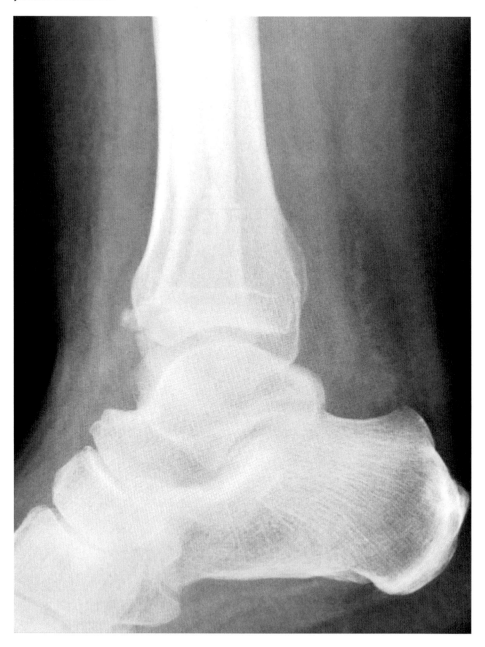

37. POISON IVY

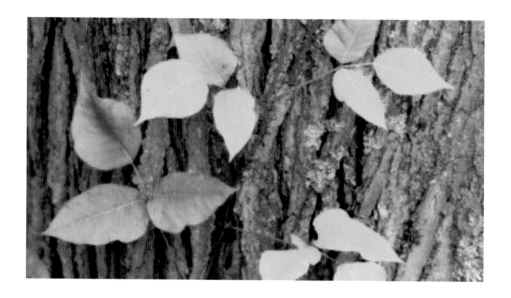

Poison Ivy plant causes an allergic reaction if you come in contact with it.

The rash causes itching, red

bumps and often lines or streaks. It needs steroid creams and allergy medicines to make the rash and itching better.

You will need to wash and wipe down everything that may have touched oil of the plant to make sure your skin does not get in contact with it again.

Fun Fact :

Poison Ivy plants are not actually poisonous.

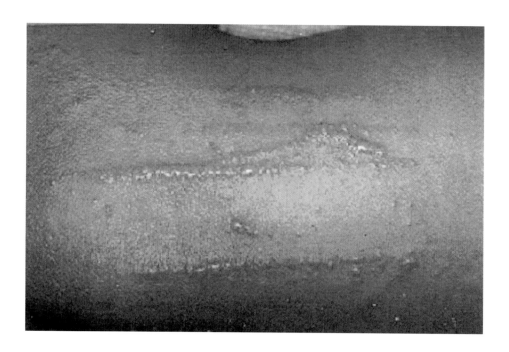

38. HERNIA

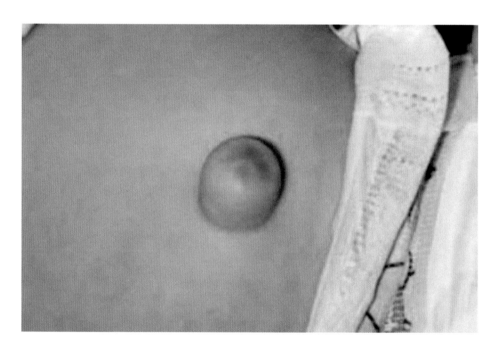

A hernia is a hole in the muscle wall.

One of the most common types of hernia is the Belly button hernia also called umbilical hernia. The body part coming out can be pushed back but the only way to treat a hernia is by putting a patch of mesh to fix the hole.

Fun Fact :

Some babies are born with a hernia but it is not painful unless it becomes twisted.

40. SWIMMER'S EARS

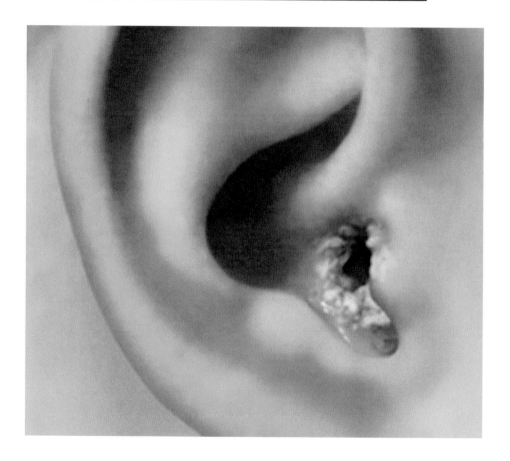

Swimmer's ear is an ear infection caused by water remaining inside the ear canal. It causes pain, redness, and swelling in the ear. Generally this will heal on its own, but occassionally you may need antibiotic drops to put in the ear. You should avoid swimming until the infection is better.

41. HEAD LICE

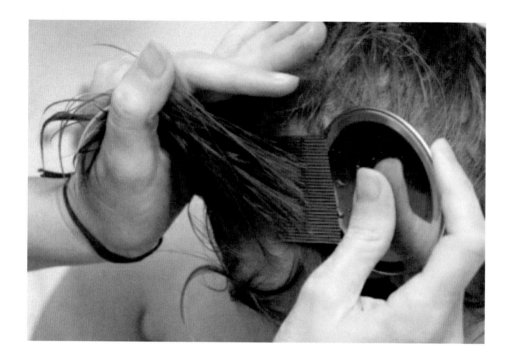

Lice can cause extreme itching in the scalp and spread from head to head. The lice feed themselves on blood but do not worry, they are not vampires.

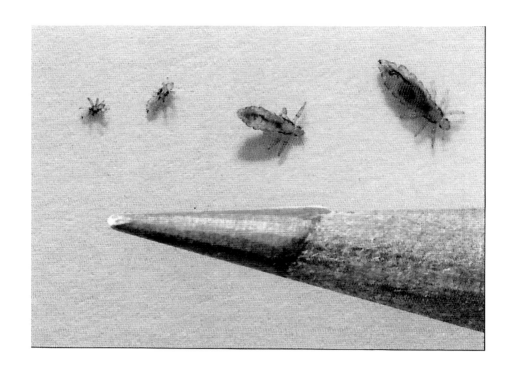

Fun Fact : Lice forms nits in the hair and scalp. Sometimes you have to shave your head to get rid of them.

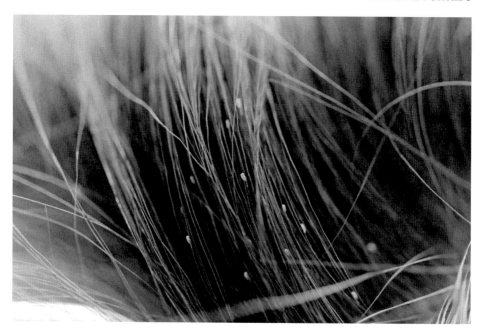

42. SCABIES

The mite Sarcoptes scabiei causes scabies. The mite lives on the skin and hatches eggs. Mostly people will have a very itchy rash in between fingers, hands, wrists.

Fun Fact : Scabies mite can only survive human skin and lives in the skin in burrows.

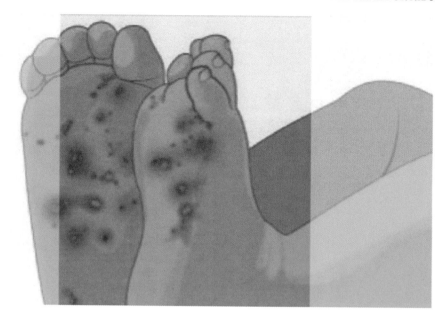

43. FOREIGN BODIES

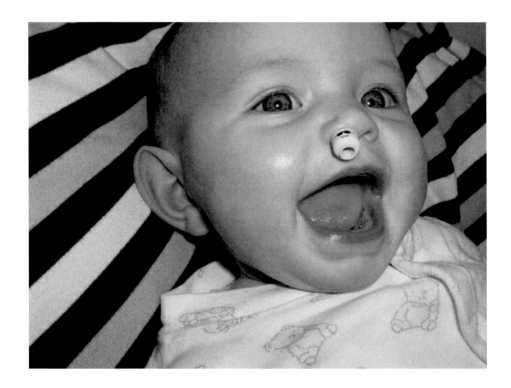

Children often put things like
peas, small toys, and pieces
of cotton inside their nose

or ears. A lego piece from the nose can be taken out with an alligator forceps (as shown)

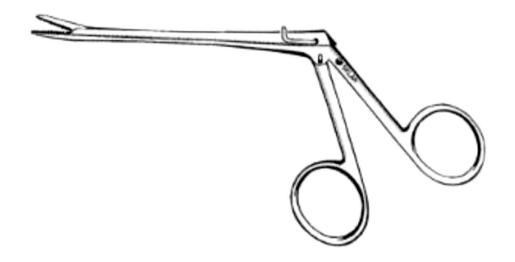

Fun Fact :

If you swallow a foreign body such as a lego piece, it may take upto 2 days for it to be pooped out!

44. INGROWN TOENAILS

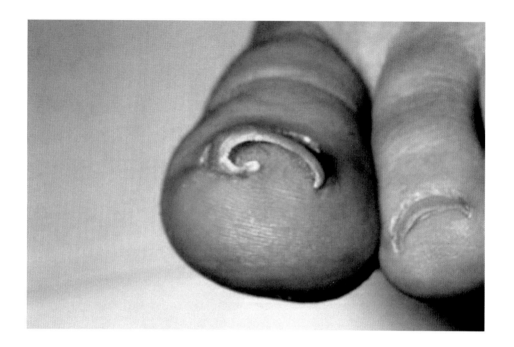

Ingrown nails occur when the corners or edges of your nail grow inside the skin that sits next to the nail. The big toe is most commonly involved. The ingrown toenails may need to have surgery to cut the edge of the nail that is digging into the skin. If your shoes do not fit you well, that may cause ingrown nail.

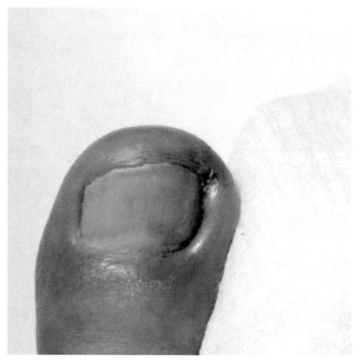

Fun Fact :

You do not have feelings of

pain in your nails or hair.
That is why you can cut them
without feeling any pain.

45. CORNEAL ABRASIONS

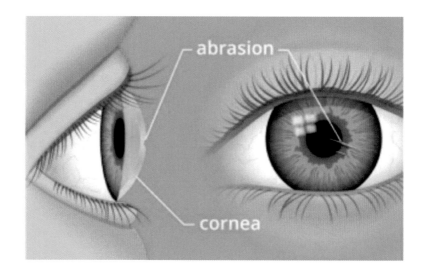

The cornea is the outer layer
over your eyes. A corneal abrasion is a scratch on the cornea
that causes severe pain and red-

ness. The person affected by a corneal abrasion becomes sensitive to light and it becomes painful to open eyes in sunlight. To check for the abrasion, the cornea is stained with fluorescein dye. The eye is than viewed under blue light to glimpse the corneal abrasion.

Fun Fact : You do not need to wear an eyepatch like a pirate if you have a corneal abrasion.

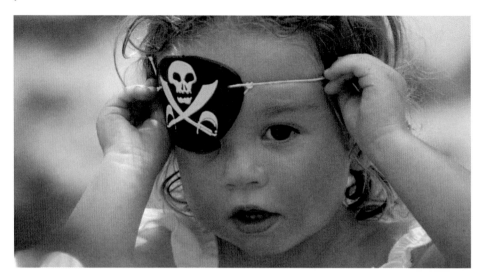

ABOUT THE AUTHOR

Jibran Naseer

Jibran resides in Illinois with his wife Sarah and their 3 young kids. He has been a practicing physician since 2008. He enjoys spending time with his chidlren and wonderful wife, teaching them about different medical scenarios. He is also a car aficionado and loves to keep up with the latest Martin Scorcese films.

Made in the USA
Middletown, DE
23 September 2021